The Star Plan

Echo Glenn

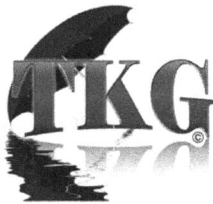

The Star Plan

First Edition © Copyright Aug 2020

Worldwide Rights Reserved
The Americas Canada Mexico Europe Asia Africa United Kingdom Finland Denmark
Northern Ireland Scotland Wales Sweden Switzerland Italy Spain Portugal Germany
Greece Austria Norway Poland Australia New Zealand China Hong Kong Japan
Singapore Philippines India Israel Ukraine Soviet Union Gulf Nations
Ashland Pismo Beach Coos Bay Grants Pass Venus Mars Jupiter Pluto Moon

Author, Echo Glenn

Editor-in-Chief, Steve William Laible, MBA

Published by The Kodel Group, LLC
P.O. Box 38, Grants Pass, Oregon, USA 97528
KodelEmpire.com

Library of Congress Control Number: 2020944433
Print ISBN-13: 978-1-62485-058-5
eBook ISBN-13: 978-1-62485-059-2

Printed in the United States of America, Europe, Asia, and beyond...

Dedication

Kippy, R.D.

Harvard Medical School Graduate
(Brigham & Women's Hospital)
(UC Davis undergrad)

"The best and most beautiful things in the world cannot be seen or even touched - they must be felt with the heart." –**Helen Keller**

Preface

Thank you for believing in yourself.

This is going to be a fun! You have to believe in the process. It will work for you.

Let the Star Plan guide you. Let the Star Plan challenge you. Let the Star Plan inspire you.

Most of all let the Star Plan shift your stars. The results will of course vary as everyone will tailor their Plan uniquely. That said if you put in the effort, the results can be splendid or magnificent.

"Do not go where the path may lead, go instead where there is no path and leave a trail."
Ralph Waldo Emerson

Monday, Monday

You must begin the Star Plan on a Monday. This gives you time to digest the material, buy or create your affirmation and achievement stars and think long and hard about your self-imposed, mandated consequences.

No matter when you receive your Star Plan book, you mustn't start until Monday. You need to get your mind around this journey. Your inner peace, balance and vibrations of the universe require it.

Silly, Silly Plan

At times this plan may seem silly. Frankly, it is. Sometimes it's the simplest things that work best. The Star Plan taps into your trust issues. Trust yourself.

If you don't trust yourself, you're going to have to let us teach you how to trust yourself. Results will dominate the day and build your trust. Believe in the day.

KISS Theory

The Star Plan is an innovate approach that tests your true resolve. Utilizing the KISS Theory [Keep it Simple Stupid] this plan could not be simpler. How well you adhere to the Star Plan will dramatically affect your results. You may not improvise. You must follow orders. Can you do that?

The basic principle is positive reinforcement which will change your behavior. Food is not the enemy, your brain is. It's not *what* you eat inasmuch as it is 'how much you eat.'

You can eat this much: [   ]

NOT this much: [   ]

Make sense?

In fact, you can eat basically anything you want. You have to know, it's about *portion control* more than any one thing.

It's also about the time it takes to consumer whatever it is you're eating. We're going to slow that down for you. As we load our own plates, we always pile it on. Is it any wonder then how 'packing it on' is manifested?

We need to feed 'hunger' not emotions. Let that sink in for a moment. You need to feed hunger not emotions. You must be mindful not mindless when it comes to your consumption levels.

You will be delighted with the results. Play the game. Have fun. You will not be sorry. Enjoy. Savor. Celebrate.

Positive Reinforcement

Many of us were molded in our early development adolescence with some sort of positive reinforcement in some fashion or another. Maybe it was a trophy, a monetary incentive (an allowance), school grades on daily or weekly homework papers, tests and report cards, merit badges, pins, or some other recognition feature.

The Star Plan taps in to that Achievement/Reward/Recognition/muscle memory. Much like a chiropractor aligns your spine or how a good massage works to relieve stress or kinks from your tired body, the Star Plan endeavors to realign your spirit, self-esteem, and self-confidence, while having a little fun in the meantime.

For many of us growing up, we had recognition or achievement gold stars in class. We're going to tap into that dormant positive reinforcement memory bank and bring you back to life. Stat!

This book is meant to improve your physical appearance but more importantly, improve your inside health and overall well-being. You will also help stimulate the economy because you're going to need a whole new wardrobe sister. (Men too.)

Life is simply too short to carry extra pounds that weigh us down, leads to disease, medical expenses and a lower quality of life. This plan folds exercise into your routine quite nicely. It's not what you expect or imagine. That's going to be a little surprise for you later in the material.

Measurements

You need more than pounds on a scale or inches gained (or lost) to document your progress. Besides, there are variables in those calculations.

Did you step on your scales in exactly the same place at the exact same time? Were you wearing exactly the same thing? Did you wait to cleanse your bowels first? Did you fudge a little knowing full well if you placed your heels or toes on the scales at a different location (not the sweet spot) or do you teeter back and forth trying to shave a pound or two from the dial? We all do it. It's not like I was watching you through a two-way mirror or anything.

Did you loop that tape around your body parts precisely as you did before? You need a much more pronounced and accurate daily reinforcement ladder—a better visual, if you will.

Within 90 days you will be strong enough (willpower wise) to secure the life you want! You will be in total control of food rather than it being in total control of you. You will be fully capable of continuing on this path all on your own. #StarsShifted

As an FYI, you might care to download the Kindle version of this book which is in color. (If you have a Kindle Unlimited Membership, it's FREE!) Print those pages where color stars, illustrations, logos or charts exist. You can then print them on temporary sticky (label) sheets to cut, peel & paste for placement on your daily Star Calendar.

STAR POWER

"The size of your success is measured by the strength of your desire; the size of your dream; and how you handle disappointment along the way."

~Robert Kiyosaki

The four stars you will be using are blue, green, silver and gold. These stars are significant and independent in their own right yet interconnected to your overall success.

[This assumes you are not colorblind. If this is case, use numbers.]

Blue is the good star.

Green, not so much.

Silver is a milestone star.

Gold is of course, the gold standard.

Blue Stars

Blue Stars represent your daily affirmations! A successful day is when you were able to completely ignore and avoid consumption of any items on your Green Star list.

It's up to you to pick a Blue Star at the beginning of every day that best represents what you're 'feeling' and post it to your calendar.

Placing the Blue Star on your calendar every morning is important. It establishes the beginning of the new you. It's not about you being worried or hungry or anything defeatist, negative or catastrophic. It's about projecting—positive thoughts about your day and coaching yourself to victory!

Green Stars

These are the dreaded stars meant to alert you that you are considering or have already consumed an item(s) from the Green Star list. A list that *you* devised.

Now, this can be problematic if Green is your favorite color. I suppose, just this once, you may improvise by making your Green Stars the Good Stars and another color the Bad Stars. Maybe Red?

[I once attended my mother's 10 year high school class reunion—a hot summer picnic in a beautiful park. Someone had brought this horrible *green* jello dish with carrot shavings, shredded coconut and other unimaginable things like raisins. It was putrid. Hence, GREEN is my childhood color of great despair. Though, only a specific shade of green turns my stomach. Green eyes are beautiful, as long as I don't have to eat one.]

Each week, you may modify, edit, and revise your Green Star list by adding to it or deleting items or clarifying portions, but not during the week, not once you've started.

It is important to establish for the week the Green Star list that is important to you. You can be strict or lenient on yourself. This is your Star Plan.

Example of a Green Star List
(List must be attached near your calendar.)
The Refrigerator Door is Ideal.

Oath

"I will not eat cookies, cakes, candy, chips, crackers, cheese, pizzas, pastries, pudding, pies, ice cream, chocolate, butter, bread, pasta, this week—Includes tapioca, cupcakes, peanut butter, licorice."

Devise your personal Green Star list with your own challenging food items. Test yourself. Maybe go slow. Those which you know are a weakness.

Perhaps include: soda pop (even diet), fruit juices, liquor, beer, wine, candy, nuts, second helpings or whatever else you want or need help with. You are going into battle.

You may most certainly specify a specific number for the week as an example.

"I will not eat more than one (1) cookie, (1) bite or slice of cake, (1) candy, (5) chips, (7) crackers, (1) oz of cheese, (2) pizza slices, (1) pastry, (1) bite of pudding, (2) bites of pies, (2) bites of ice cream, etc., bread, pasta, this week— Includes tapioca, cupcakes, peanut butter, licorice for the entire week. And I will NOT cram a mouthful of anything as I will be using my very own special consumption spoon."

19

Your Green Star list will not be identical every week or exactly the same as your challenge partner's. That's okay. Maybe you begin with one item or two or three. #KissTheory

Green Star

Consequences Chart

You must determine your own consequences. We have provided some examples. If you go easy on yourself, you won't have the necessary motivation that is required to force behavior modification or what you're trying to discover in yourself.

It's assured if you do this plan with someone in your household, spouse, neighbor, co-worker, social media, or best friend, your accountability is far more realistic—and it sets off a little healthy competition—one more layer of incentives. It's just too easy to fake it or not follow through when you're only accountable to yourself. Make sense? So, get creative. It's sort of akin to Truth or Dare.

Truth or Dare

You must sit down and over the next few days and determine your consequences for every Green Star you place on your calendar. It ought to cost you dearly.

Your consequences must be outside your comfort zone. Maybe if you are doing this with a partner or in a group, you can all arrive at the appropriate consequences. They don't have to be in any particular order but it helps if you do show progression in severity. This certainly isn't about fat shaming you or embarrassing you. It's about waking you up.

It's about lessons you learned in your childhood. It's okay to bully yourself!

In fact, it is recommended you create your new Green Star List of items on Sunday afternoon for the upcoming week.

Green Star Consequences

Back to those dreaded consequences. Beyond placing your Green Stars on your calendar, you will also now have to fulfill your consequences. It's a mandatory requirement. It's not meant as a punishment. This is just you honoring the commitment you made to yourself before you began this endeavor. You must honor yourself. Perform your consequence within 24 hours. Rain or shine. If you placed a Green Star on Monday then you have until Tuesday; if you placed a

2nd Green Star on Tuesday, you have until Wednesday to fulfill your consequence.

Monday, you will begin anew. Monday's are always a fresh start day. Nobody expects you to fly through the week unscathed. Trust the process. Eventually, your calendar will reveal no Green Stars. Nothing but Blue, Silver and Gold stars!

Each week you are allowed to adjust your Green Star list. If you have to make it easier for yourself, then do that. If you want to challenge yourself for the upcoming week, then do that.

The Green Star represents those food items you need help avoiding or limiting. Make sure you keep a copy of every Green Star list. You'll want to look back and assess your reasoning or bargaining with yourself.

Have fun with this. Once it's on your list you are not permitted to remove it from your list until the following week.

So be thoughtful when placing items on your Green Star list you are willing to forego (or limit) for the week.

If you simply cannot resist an item, you will pay the consequence—that's known as a negative reinforcement and trust me, it works!! It works only if you're honest with yourself. You are not permitted to rationalize or make excuses at any point during this process. You will NOT bargain with yourself. That's a mindset we have to break. Take responsibility. It's a special occasion; it's a birthday party; I deserve it; it's a one-time thing; I'm hungry; I forgot it was on my list; No one will know, the dog ate my cupcake, etc. Knock it off. Don't do that. Don't lie to yourself.

Trust

The Star Plan trusts you to complete your Sunday without consuming any items on the Green Star list.

This is a leap of faith. But it also puts the responsibility on you to behave. It adds yet another layer or barrier to protect you from yourself. You would have to put a Green Star over top of your Gold Star and look at that every day. You will also have 24 hours to perform your consequence. You really want to get to where you are not having any consequences in your life.

Well, any Star Plan consequences that is. As you are tempted, you will have to *weigh* the consequence. Is it worth it?

Consequences are meant to keep you on track—a moment on the lips, a lifetime on the hips—but a very clean neighborhood at that. These moats will protect you from yourself—eventually.

If after earning five Blue Stars (Monday through Friday) and earning a Saturday Silver Star, it's a calculated assumption you wouldn't dare jeopardize earning your Gold Star on Sunday mornings.

While the Star Plan trusts you! You must also trust the Star Plan and yourself. This is about honesty, self-worth, and integrity. *Doing the right thing even if no one is watching!*

If by some fall from grace you succumb to temptation and consume an item on your Green Star list during the day or night, you are required to place a Green Star on your calendar on top of any previous placed Gold or Silver Stars.

This also does not mean you can now open the flood gates and binge. It simply means you are a work in progress. You will do better the next week.

Or donate your Star Plan book to Goodwill and be done with it.

Off to find yet another 'diet' plan.

Just remember, YOU are the common denominator here.

Green Star Consequence
Example No. 1

You must wash a neighbor's car the very first time you post a Green Star.

Your conversation dialogue is as follows: "Hi Stan. I busted my Star Plan and now my self-imposed consequence is to wash your car. Where's your hose?"

You must accomplish this task within 24 hours clearing the slate for a fresh start.

Green Star Consequence
Example No. 2

The 2nd time you post a Green Star on your calendar, you must wash a stranger's car. This will raise your stress level and teach you a valuable lesson.

At every stage your consequences must grow more challenging. More demanding of yourself.

Green Star Consequence Example No. 3

The 3rd time you post a Green Star, you must … Wash your own widows, a neighbor's windows, mow your lawn, or mow a neighbor's lawn or rake leaves or whatever it is you want to test yourself with by giving yourself a truly rewarding and challenging task to get your mind right. Maybe you just stand on a street corner for 30 minutes with a sandwich board or sign stating how you are working the Star Plan.

That's all your sign needs to read. "I am working the Star Plan."

This isn't SEAL training. This is way more difficult than that.

The key here is not to beat yourself up but do be creative and make sure you have given yourself some incentive for NOT consuming a tasty item on the Green Star list. Do not Green Star yourself.

Post your Consequences to Facebook. Let the world know how you are Green Starring yourself. Be as elaborate as you must to affect change.

Maybe you're shy. Then make your Green Star Consequence something that is opposite of that. Something that will give you pause the next time you want to treat yourself to a Green Star item. Walk up to a stranger at Costco and look them square in the eyes and tell them you are from one of the five Pluto moons, or the Planet Neptune or Uranus or Saturn. Or strike up an uncomfortable conversation. Tell them one of the items in their cart is on your Green Star list. That ought to do it.

Better yet, if you are doing the Star Plan with someone, devise consequences that are not for you but the other person. Be forewarned, you will be subject to their consequence for you too.

This is where it gets fun and serious. You must honor the consequences you set. Otherwise, you just wasted your money for this book.

Ideally, a wonderful, painless even, consequence is to just donate $5 to the global Star Plan contingency fund at:

PayPal.me/thekodelgroup

You can save the embarrassment and shame by making a philanthropic gesture of goodwill instead. #CampTenderheart

Silver Stars

Silver Stars are placed on your calendar only on Saturday mornings after you've completed Monday through Friday with nothing but Blue Stars.

In other words, no Green Stars!

A Silver Star is a well-earned, well-deserved echelon achievement award for enjoying an entire Blue Star week. If you have even one Green Star on your calendar you have not earned your Silver Star. You must wait for next week and begin again.

It takes a solid week, Monday through Friday of Blue Stars to earn your Saturday Silver Star and only after those brilliant 6 days do you earn your Gold Star! But wait...

Gold Stars

On Sunday mornings, if you have avoided those items on your Green Star list through Saturday midnight, you have earned the coveted Gold Star.

Place a much deserved Gold Star on your calendar as early as Saturday at midnight or on Sunday morning when you awake. This is a little reward incentive; a treat to propel you through Sunday before you've even made it through that day yet.

It says, "I believe in you. You can do this. I trust you. There is NO WAY you will consume any Green Star items today! There is no way you will want to put a Green Star over your Gold Star." That is a visual no one wants to see.

For every Green Star list item you consume you must place Green Stars on your calendar for that day. This is not meant to shame you but rather document your behavior, willpower and progress.

Some of you will invariably have 1-2 Green Stars on any given day. That at least identifies where you need work. Lessen your Green Star list items. Make it easier on yourself. This isn't about self-sabotage. Better to be way more realistic. #BabySteps

It is not uncommon to have a rather colorful calendar those first few weeks. That is until you buy-in to wanting to do better.

The fact that you have fallen off the proverbial wagon is just a sign that you need the Star Plan more than you first realized.

Baby Steps

You will be required to replace your utensils (fork and spoon) with a baby spoon.

You are allowed to use a knife (as opposed to your finger or thumb) to help slide food onto your new consumption device. But that's really not going to be a problem as you will learn. Gerber makes their baby spoons in different colored soft tips so purchase a few. A pink spoon can be for regular meals during the week and a purple baby spoon can be for special occasions.

By reducing the size of your 'face shovel' you will slow your roll. It's called 'mindful' eating. It's a great way to slow your pace.

Shoveling your food mindlessly is a common mistake and increases your calorie count immensely. Slowing down your hand to mouth cadence and function will give you more pleasure to enjoy your meals. It also gives you time for your brain to alert you that you are maybe not full but are satiated.

A cup of yogurt will now take you five minutes to consume rather than 90 seconds. A bowl of soup will take you a full week. ☺ As will a bowl of cereal. And forget about a salad. Those leaves won't stay on that spoon no matter what. The plan entices you to savor your food. You'll be surprised at how much fun it is. One macaroni noodle per baby spoon will get your attention!

Portion control is a critical factor in keeping you healthy. There's something called your 'inside' health. It's the most important part of being healthy. Not to get too wonky but as your blood sugar rises, it's like gumming up a keyhole so your cells can't perform their function.

A more drastic illustration of what high blood sugar does is it's like shards of glass destroying your veins, arteries, organs.

The tiniest of blood vessels in your eye can be severely damaged. So before you let your eyes deceive you about that tasty morsel you're about to consume, it's equally important to understand the long-term, continued, conditioned, damaging consequences of to your inside health.

Inventory

These are the items you will need:

1. Baby Spoon(s)
2. Blue Stars

3. Green Stars

4. Silver Stars

5. Gold Stars

6. Calendar

7. Green Star List

8. Stated Consequence(s)

RECAP No. 1

The first thing you must do is take an inventory of all those tempting delights you have in your pantry, purse, desk, secret hiding stash, that you know in your heart adds weight to your butt, hips, waist, neck, thighs, arms, legs and face.

You can begin the Star Plan slowly or abruptly. It's entirely up to you. But once you start, you must behave.

Devise your Green Star List and your stated Consequences.

RECAP No. 2

You must follow the rules. If you're not a rules follower by nature, indulge the plan. You can always return to your life in search of yet another solution later.

If you deviate in any way, shape or form, you're not benefiting from this book.

See if you can find anyone who wants to do this with you. Explain the Plan Stan.

Get your Calendar and put it on the refrigerator door or some other place but it should be in plain view if not living alone.

Might be wise to dispose of any items on that Green Star list. I'm just sayin'...

RECAP No. 3

The most important thing here is not to give up. If you post a Green Star, it's not the end of the world. It's a *hiccup* in your week. You get back on that horse the very next day.

RECAP No. 4

Charting

By charting your daily progress *honestly* you will begin seeing a string of Stars. If those are Blue Stars, you so got this. If however, they are Green Stars, you're going to have to sit down and reflect on why this is happening. Give yourself a full week before you pivot.

If you must begin again and again and again until you get it right, then do that.

A lifetime of poor or chronic eating habits will be smack dab in your face far beyond any rationales, excuses or deal-making with your mind. We are going to help you replace those cravings, urgings with a better, stronger achievement reinforced reward—safely. Cold Turkey!

Just kidding. Yes, it is akin to cold turkey but it's actually replacing the *momentary* taste bud satisfaction with an imprinted memorialized calendar of recognition and achievement and reward that will serve as building blocks changing how you see food. Your Star Calendar will be with you as a constant daily reminder speaking to you. A visual STAR satisfaction is longer lasting. It is our belief, earning those stars are going to become your escape.

Crossroads

Losing weight is actually a byproduct of the plan. The weight reduction you experience is a positive *consequence* for your good behavior. The Star Plan helps you take back your power both psychologically and physiologically.

If you also post your weekly calendar on Facebook for instance, you will not only be helping others but reinforcing your own efforts. It's really just another way of journaling but with a visual pat on the back. Whose the good boy, whose the good boy? ☺

Ivan Petrovich Pavlov, founder of modern behavior therapy, was a Russian physiologist known primarily for his work in classical conditioning. **This is that.**

You will be at a crossroads in the beginning. Should I eat this or reward myself with a STAR. It might seem trivial or trite in the beginning, but make no mistake, eventually the STARS win out.

44

That's going to be your tipping point, especially as you begin stringing Blue, then Silver then Gold Stars together, week after week. You are in effect, shifting your stars. The visualization becomes even more powerful as behavior modification creates its own synergy.

Think Beyond the Act

You must condition yourself or learn to 'Think Beyond the Act.' If you choose an action that commands a Green Star, you must own it. It's as simple as that. Puking does not resolve you. You must still pay the piper—a Green Star on your Star Calendar and a Consequence. No bargaining here. You must do the time as it were. It's a delightful way of looking at yourself in ways you've likely never had to do before.

Your character is at play here—your integrity.

"Life begins at the end of your comfort zone."
Neale Donald Walsch

Recapping: You will need to construct your own consequences chart before you begin the Star Plan. Pick things that make you uncomfortable.

Every time you post a Green Star to your daily Star Calendar, you must implement your consequence. Be brave. This is your own doing. You must take responsibility.

I hope that 'cake' was worth it.

Just as those dreaded Green Stars play a vital role in the Star Plan, as has been the focus of this book, so do the Blue Stars.

Let's NEVER forget the Blue Stars.

Daily Affirmations

(Positive Words)

"Hugs can do great amounts of good, especially for children."
Diana, Princess of Wales

How about you also give yourself a daily hug! Do it with affirmations. Put these words on your Star Plan, at least daily but hourly if need be. Give yourself permission to love yourself. You are going to love yourself, once and for all, no matter your weight. This is an empirical truth.

WRITE AT LEAST ONE AFFIRMATION WORD A DAY ON YOUR DAILY

STAR CALENDAR

We've also put them on your Blue Stars if you'd rather print and paste. You will need to get a Kindle Version for the color.

A. A-OK adorable ace awesome astute ablaze appealing alluring appealing admirable affable agreeable amusing admired adored accepting attractive

B. beautiful blue-ribbon blue-chip brilliant blazing bold best brilliance booming beloved blessed blissful beaming

C. cool clarity consummate cloud nine champion crowned cherished captivating charming cheerful cordial calming candescent cute

D. dandy divine delightful dazzling delighted desirable darling delectable delicious dreamy dapper

E. empowered exemplary excellent exceptional eminence ecstatic euphoric elated extraordinary endearing engaging enchanting entrancing enjoyable enviable empathic eye-catching elegant exquisite excitement

F. first-rate first-class far out fab fantastic fabulous faithful faultless flawless faultless flourishing flowering favored favorite fascinating fetching friendly flattered flattering foxy

G. gleaming groovy great glorious greatness glowing gangbusters growth gracious grateful good gorgeous glamorous

H. healthy honored heavenly handsome hot hunky

I. incredible impressive inviting impeccable immaculate illuminated incandescent

J. jubilant joyful jolly

K. kissable kind knockout

L. lovely luminous lustrous love life
lovesome loveable loved likeable luscious

M. magnificent magic marvelous

N. nice neat nirvanic noble nifty

O. outstanding overjoyed over the moon

P. perfect peerless prime peachy pristine
pretty picture-perfect promising precious
pleasant pleasing pleasurable pleasant
personable praiseful

Q. quintessential queenly quiddity quiet

R. remarkable radiant rapturous roaring
robust respect respected relished ravishing

S. supreme superlative splendid sweet smart
superior superb swell sensational super
second to none spotless superiority shining

smile shimmering socko satisfying soothing
sparkling supportive sympathetic stunning
show-stopping snazzy striking seductive
sexy studly suave stylish

T. terrific tremendous top-notch true thrilled
triumphant thriving treasured tasty tempting

U. unbeatable unsurpassed ultimate
unrivaled unequaled unparalleled

V. vivid vivacious valiant validatory vaulted

W. wicked good whew wonderful without
equal winning winsome warm

X. xanthic xenial xenogenic

Y. youthful yummy yams

Z. zingy zestful zen zany zappy zazzy

BLUE STAR
(Affirmations)

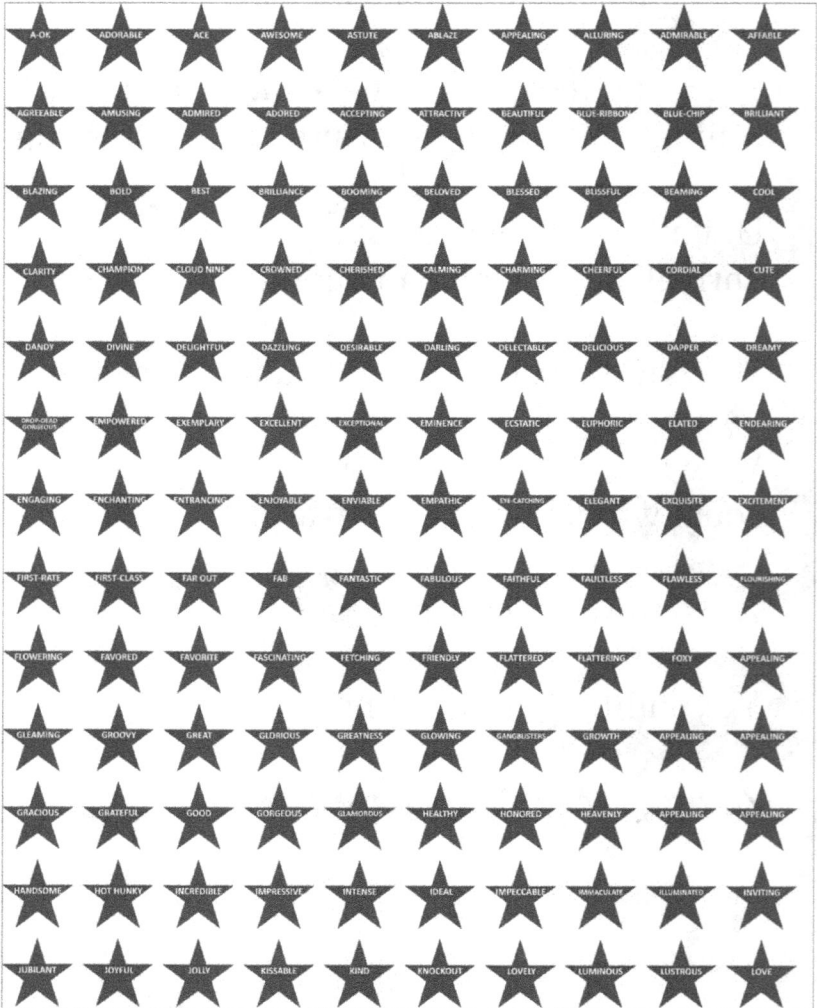

A-OK	ADORABLE	ACE	AWESOME	ASTUTE	ABLAZE	APPEALING	ALLURING	ADMIRABLE	AFFABLE
AGREEABLE	AMUSING	ADMIRED	ADORED	ACCEPTING	ATTRACTIVE	BEAUTIFUL	BLUE-RIBBON	BLUE-CHIP	BRILLIANT
BLAZING	BOLD	BEST	BRILLIANCE	BOOMING	BELOVED	BLESSED	BLISSFUL	BEAMING	COOL
CLARITY	CHAMPION	CLOUD NINE	CROWNED	CHERISHED	CALMING	CHARMING	CHEERFUL	CORDIAL	CUTE
DANDY	DIVINE	DELIGHTFUL	DAZZLING	DESIRABLE	DARLING	DELECTABLE	DELICIOUS	DAPPER	DREAMY
DROP-DEAD GORGEOUS	EMPOWERED	EXEMPLARY	EXCELLENT	EXCEPTIONAL	EMINENCE	ECSTATIC	EUPHORIC	ELATED	ENDEARING
ENGAGING	ENCHANTING	ENTRANCING	ENJOYABLE	ENVIABLE	EMPATHIC	EYE-CATCHING	ELEGANT	EXQUISITE	EXCITEMENT
FIRST-RATE	FIRST-CLASS	FAR OUT	FAB	FANTASTIC	FABULOUS	FAITHFUL	FAULTLESS	FLAWLESS	FLOURISHING
FLOWERING	FAVORED	FAVORITE	FASCINATING	FETCHING	FRIENDLY	FLATTERED	FLATTERING	FOXY	APPEALING
GLEAMING	GROOVY	GREAT	GLORIOUS	GREATNESS	GLOWING	GANGBUSTERS	GROWTH	APPEALING	APPEALING
GRACIOUS	GRATEFUL	GOOD	GORGEOUS	GLAMOROUS	HEALTHY	HONORED	HEAVENLY	APPEALING	APPEALING
HANDSOME	HOT HUNKY	INCREDIBLE	IMPRESSIVE	INTENSE	IDEAL	IMPECCABLE	IMMACULATE	ILLUMINATED	INVITING
JUBILANT	JOYFUL	JOLLY	KISSABLE	KIND	KNOCKOUT	LOVELY	LUMINOUS	LUSTROUS	LOVE

"Don't judge each day by the harvest you reap but by the seeds that you plant."
–Robert Louis Stevenson

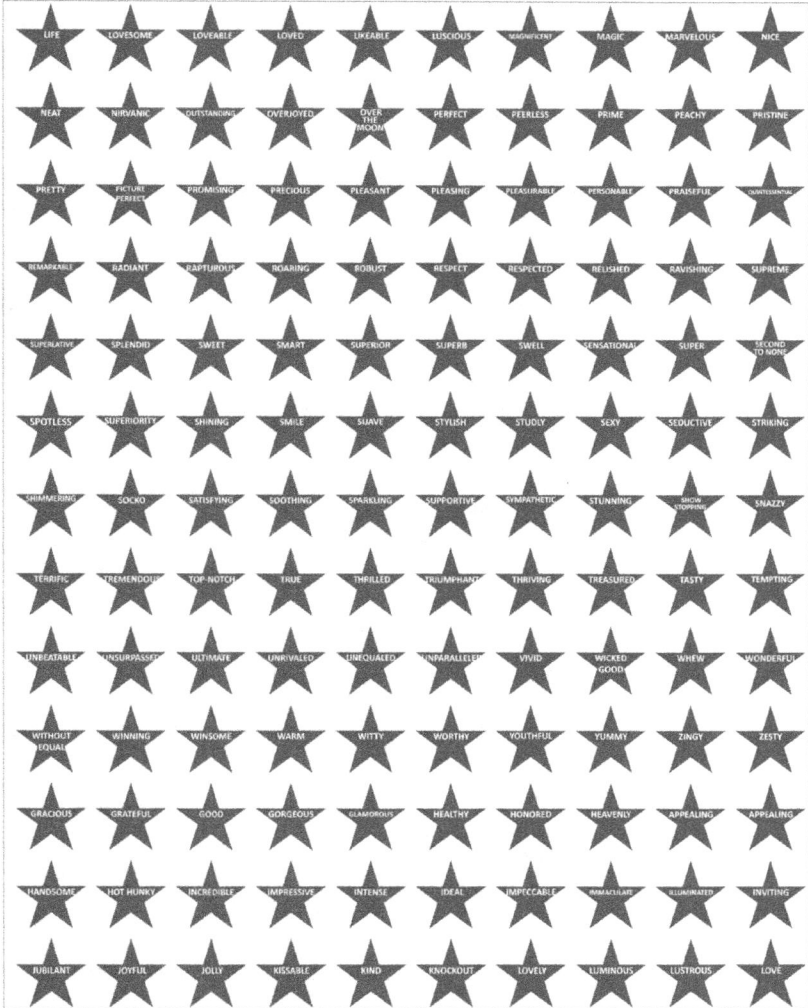

LIFE	LOVESOME	LOVEABLE	LOVED	LIKEABLE	LUSCIOUS	MAGNIFICENT	MAGIC	MARVELOUS	NICE
NEAT	NIRVANIC	OUTSTANDING	OVERJOYED	OVER THE MOON	PERFECT	PEERLESS	PRIME	PEACHY	PRISTINE
PRETTY	PICTURE PERFECT	PROMISING	PRECIOUS	PLEASANT	PLEASING	PLEASURABLE	PERSONABLE	PRAISEFUL	QUINTESSENTIAL
REMARKABLE	RADIANT	RAPTUROUS	ROARING	ROBUST	RESPECT	RESPECTED	RELISHED	RAVISHING	SUPREME
SUPERLATIVE	SPLENDID	SWEET	SMART	SUPERIOR	SUPERB	SWELL	SENSATIONAL	SUPER	SECOND TO NONE
SPOTLESS	SUPERIORITY	SHINING	SMILE	SUAVE	STYLISH	STUDLY	SEXY	SEDUCTIVE	STRIKING
SHIMMERING	SOCKO	SATISFYING	SOOTHING	SPARKLING	SUPPORTIVE	SYMPATHETIC	STUNNING	SHOW STOPPING	SNAZZY
TERRIFIC	TREMENDOUS	TOP-NOTCH	TRUE	THRILLED	TRIUMPHANT	THRIVING	TREASURED	TASTY	TEMPTING
UNBEATABLE	UNSURPASSED	ULTIMATE	UNRIVALED	UNEQUALED	UNPARALLELED	VIVID	WICKED GOOD	WHEW	WONDERFUL
WITHOUT EQUAL	WINNING	WINSOME	WARM	WITTY	WORTHY	YOUTHFUL	YUMMY	ZINGY	ZESTY
GRACIOUS	GRATEFUL	GOOD	GORGEOUS	GLAMOROUS	HEALTHY	HONORED	HEAVENLY	APPEALING	APPEALING
HANDSOME	HOT HUNKY	INCREDIBLE	IMPRESSIVE	INTENSE	IDEAL	IMPECCABLE	IMMACULATE	ILLUMINATED	INVITING
JUBILANT	JOYFUL	JOLLY	KISSABLE	KIND	KNOCKOUT	LOVELY	LUMINOUS	LUSTROUS	LOVE

Gender Logos
Use the appropriate gender logo on your calendar.

★ The Star Plan © 2017 The Kodel Group, LLC - PO Box 38, Grants Pass, Oregon 97528 - info@kodelgroup.com

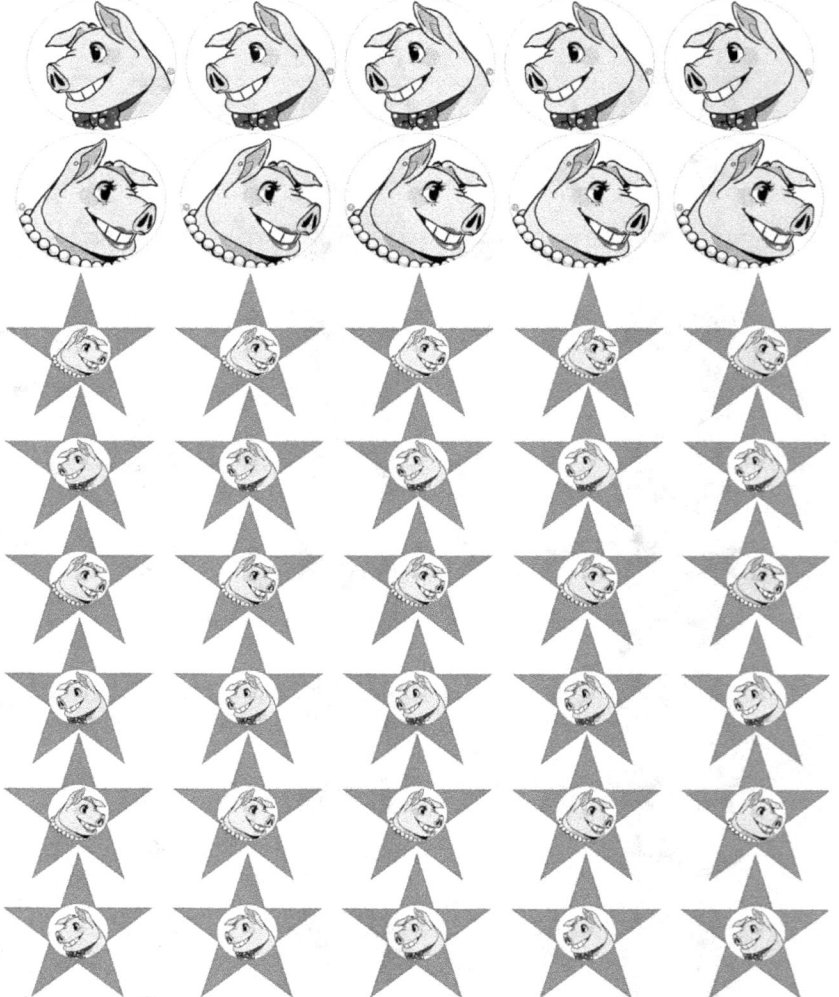

★ The Star Plan © 2017 The Kodel Group, LLC - PO Box 38, Grants Pass, Oregon 97528 - info@kodelgroup.com

GOLD & SILVER STARS

Star Calendar
You must begin on a Monday
(Regardless of the date)

**For this example, you would begin on the
Monday of the previous month.
Your 1st week would 6 days by Saturday.**

**Saturdays are reserved for Silver Stars
Sundays are reserved for Gold Stars**

SUN	MON	TUE	WED	THU	FRI	SAT
		1	2	3	4	5
6	7	8	9	10	11	12
13	14	15	16	17	18	19
20	21	22	23	24	25	26
27	28	29	30	31		

Good Luck! Have Fun! Be Safe!

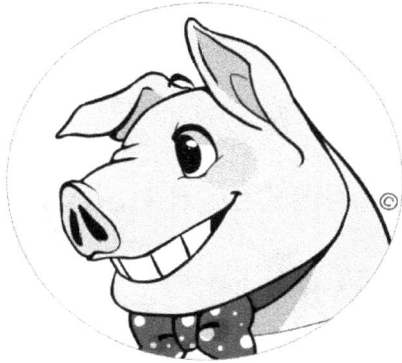

"Never love anyone who treats you
like you're ordinary."
Oscar Wilde

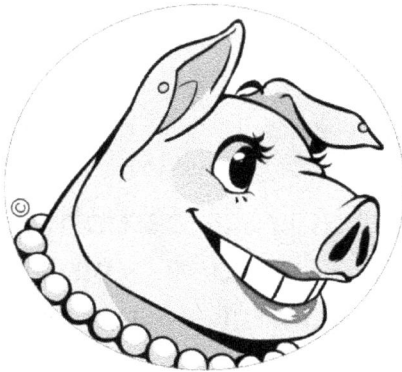

The End

Mayo Clinic

Low-carb diet: Can it help you lose weight?

Could a low-carb diet give you an edge in losing weight? Help you keep weight off permanently? Here's what you need to know about the low-carb diet.

Definition

A low-carb diet limits carbohydrates — such as those found in grains, starchy vegetables and fruit — and emphasizes foods high in protein and fat. Many types of low-carb diets exist. Each diet has varying restrictions on the types and amounts of carbohydrates you can eat.

Purpose

A low-carb diet is generally used for losing weight. Some low-carb diets may have health benefits beyond weight loss, such as reducing risk factors associated with Type 2 diabetes and metabolic syndrome.

Why you might follow a low-carb diet

You might choose to follow a low-carb diet because you:

- Want a diet that restricts certain carbs to help you lose weight

- Want to change your overall eating habits

- Enjoy the types and amounts of foods featured in low-carb diets

Check with your doctor before starting any weight-loss diet, especially if you have any health conditions, such as diabetes or heart disease.

Diet details

As the name says, a low-carb diet restricts the type and amount of carbohydrates you eat. Carbohydrates are a type of calorie-providing macronutrient found in many foods and beverages.

Carbohydrates can be simple or complex. They can further be classified as simple refined (table sugar), simple natural (lactose in milk and fructose in fruit), complex refined (white flour) and complex natural (whole grains or beans).

Common sources of naturally occurring carbohydrates include:

- Grains
- Fruits
- Vegetables
- Milk
- Nuts
- Seeds
- Legumes (beans, lentils, peas)

Food manufacturers also add refined carbohydrates to processed foods in the form of sugar or white flour. Examples of foods that contain refined carbohydrates are white breads and pasta, cookies, cake, candy, and sugar-sweetened sodas and drinks.

Your body uses carbohydrates as its main fuel source. Complex carbohydrates (starches) are broken down into simple sugars during digestion.

They're then absorbed into your bloodstream, where they're known as blood sugar (glucose). In general, natural complex carbohydrates are digested more slowly and they have less effect on blood sugar.

Natural complex carbohydrates provide bulk and serve other body functions beyond fuel.

Rising levels of blood sugar trigger the body to release insulin. Insulin helps glucose enter your body's cells. Some glucose is used by your body for energy, fueling all of your activities, whether it's going for a jog or simply breathing. Extra glucose is usually stored in your liver, muscles and other cells for later use or is converted to fat.

The idea behind the low-carb diet is that decreasing carbs lowers insulin levels, which causes the body to burn stored fat for energy and ultimately leads to weight loss.

Typical foods for a low-carb diet

In general, a low-carb diet focuses on proteins, including meat, poultry, fish and eggs, and some non-starchy vegetables.

A low-carb diet generally excludes or limits most grains, legumes, fruits, breads, sweets, pastas and starchy vegetables, and sometimes nuts and seeds. Some low-carb diet plans allow small amounts of certain fruits, vegetables and whole grains.

A daily limit of 0.7 to 2 ounces (20 to 60 grams) of carbohydrates is typical with a low-carb diet.

These amounts of carbohydrates provide 80 to 240 calories. Some low-carb diets greatly restrict carbs during the initial phase of the diet and then gradually increase the number of allowed carbs.

In contrast, the Dietary Guidelines for Americans recommends that carbohydrates make up 45 to 65 percent of your total daily calorie intake.

So if you consume 2,000 calories a day, you would need to eat between 900 and 1,300 calories a day from carbohydrates.

Results

Weight loss

Most people can lose weight if they restrict the number of calories consumed and increase physical activity levels. To lose 1 to 1.5 pounds (0.5 to 0.7 kilogram) a week, you need to reduce your daily calories by 500 to 750 calories.

Low-carb diets, especially very low-carb diets, may lead to greater short-term weight loss than do low-fat diets. But most studies have found that at 12 or 24 months, the benefits of a low-carb diet are not very large.

A 2015 review found that higher protein, low-carbohydrate diets may offer a slight advantage in terms of weight loss and loss of fat mass compared with a normal protein diet.

Cutting calories and carbs may not be the only reason for the weight loss. Some studies show that you may shed some weight because the extra protein and fat keeps you feeling full longer, which helps you eat less.

Other health benefits

Low-carb diets may help prevent or improve serious health conditions, such as metabolic syndrome, diabetes, high blood pressure and cardiovascular disease.

In fact, almost any diet that helps you shed excess weight can reduce or even reverse risk factors for cardiovascular disease and diabetes.

Most weight-loss diets — not just low-carb diets — may improve blood cholesterol or blood sugar levels, at least temporarily.

Low-carb diets may improve high-density lipoprotein (HDL) cholesterol and triglyceride values slightly more than do moderate-carb diets.

That may be due not only to how many carbs you eat but also to the quality of your other food choices.

Lean protein (fish, poultry, legumes), healthy fats (monounsaturated and polyunsaturated) and unprocessed carbs — such as whole grains, legumes, vegetables, fruits and low-fat dairy products — are generally healthier choices.

A report from the American Heart Association, the American College of Cardiology and the Obesity Society concluded that there isn't enough evidence to say whether most low-carbohydrate diets provide heart-healthy benefits.

Risks

If you suddenly and drastically cut carbs, you may experience a variety of temporary health effects, including:

- Headache
- Bad breath
- Weakness
- Muscle cramps
- Fatigue
- Skin rash
- Constipation or diarrhea

In addition, some diets restrict carbohydrate intake so much that in the long term they can result in vitamin or mineral deficiencies, bone loss and gastrointestinal disturbances and may increase risks of various chronic diseases.

Because low-carb diets may not provide necessary nutrients, these diets aren't recommended as a method of weight loss for preteens and high schoolers.

Their growing bodies need the nutrients found in whole grains, fruits and vegetables.

Severely restricting carbohydrates to less than 0.7 ounces (20 grams) a day can result in a process called **ketosis**.

Ketosis occurs when you don't have enough sugar (glucose) for energy, so your body breaks down stored fat, causing ketones to build up in your body.

Side effects from ketosis can include nausea, headache, mental and physical fatigue, and bad breath.

It's not clear what kind of possible long-term health risks a low-carb diet may pose because most research studies have lasted less than a year.

Some health experts believe that if you eat large amounts of fat and protein from animal sources, your risk of heart disease or certain cancers may actually increase.

If you follow a low-carbohydrate diet that's higher in fat and possibly higher in protein, it's important to choose foods with healthy unsaturated fats and healthy proteins.

Limit foods containing saturated and trans fats, such as meat, high-fat dairy products, and processed crackers and pastries.

10 [Science-Backed] Reasons to Eat More Protein

Courtesy of Healthline

The health effects of fat and carbs are controversial. However, almost everyone agrees that protein is important.

Most people eat enough protein to prevent deficiency, but some individuals would do better with a much higher protein intake.

Numerous studies suggest that a high-protein diet has major benefits for weight loss and metabolic health.

Here are 10 [science-based] reasons to eat <u>more</u> protein.

1. Reduces Appetite and Hunger Levels

The three macronutrients — fats, carbs, and protein — affect your body in different ways.

Studies show that protein is by far the most filling. It helps you feel more full — with less food.

This is partly because protein reduces your level of the hunger hormone ghrelin. It also boosts the levels of peptide YY, a hormone that makes you feel full.

These effects on appetite can be powerful. In one study, increasing protein intake from 15% to 30% of calories made overweight women eat 441 fewer calories each day without intentionally restricting anything.

If you need to lose weight or belly fat, consider replacing some of your carbs and fats with protein. It can be as simple as making your potato or rice serving smaller while adding a few extra bites of meat or fish.

SUMMARY ~ A high-protein diet reduces hunger, helping you eat fewer calories. This is caused by the improved function of weight-regulating hormones.

2. Increases Muscle Mass & Strength

Protein is the building block of your muscles. Therefore, eating adequate amounts of protein helps you maintain your muscle mass and promotes muscle growth when you do strength training.

Numerous studies show that eating plenty of protein can help increase muscle muscle mass and strength.

If you're physically active, lifting weights, or trying to gain muscle, you need to make sure you're getting enough protein.

Keeping protein intake high can also help prevent muscle loss during weight loss.

SUMMARY ~ Muscle is made primarily of protein. High protein intake can help you gain muscle mass and strength while reducing muscle loss during weight loss.

3. Good for Your Bones

An ongoing myth perpetuates the idea that protein — mainly animal protein — is bad for your bones.

This is based on the idea that protein increases acid load in the body, leading to calcium leaching from your bones in order to neutralize the acid.

However, most long-term studies indicate that protein, including animal protein, has major benefits for bone health.

People who eat more protein tend to maintain bone mass better as they age and have a much lower risk of osteoporosis and fractures.

This is especially important for women, who are at high risk of osteoporosis after menopause. Eating plenty of protein and staying active is a good way to help prevent that from happening.

SUMMARY People who eat more protein tend to have **better** bone health and a much lower risk of osteoporosis and fractures as they get older.

4. Reduces Cravings and Desire for Late-Night Snacking

A food craving is different from normal hunger.

It is not just about your body needing energy or nutrients but your brain needing a reward.

Yet, cravings can be incredibly hard to control. **The best way** to overcome them may be to **prevent** them from occurring in the first place.

One of the best prevention methods is to increase your protein intake.

One study in overweight men showed that increasing protein to 25% of calories reduced cravings by 60% and the desire to snack at night by half.

Likewise, a study in overweight adolescent girls found that eating a high-protein breakfast reduced cravings and late-night snacking.

This may be mediated by an improvement in the function of dopamine, one of the main brain hormones involved in cravings and addiction.

SUMMARY Eating more protein may reduce cravings and desire for late-night snacking. Merely having a high-protein breakfast may have a powerful effect.

5. Boosts Metabolism and Increases Fat Burning

Eating can boost your metabolism for a short while.

That's because your body uses calories to digest and make use of the nutrients in foods. This is referred to as the thermic effect of food (TEF).

However, not all foods are the same in this regard. In fact, protein has a much higher thermic effect than fat or carbs — 20–35% compared to 5–15%.

High protein intake has been shown to significantly boost metabolism and increase the number of calories you burn. This can amount to 80–100 more calories burned each day.

In fact, some research suggests you can burn even more. In one study, a high-protein group burned 260 more calories per day than a low-protein group. That's equivalent to an hour of moderate-intensity exercise per day.

SUMMARY High protein intake may
boost your metabolism significantly,
helping you burn more calories
throughout the day.

6. Lowers Your Blood Pressure

High blood pressure is a major
cause of heart attacks, strokes, and
chronic kidney disease.

Interestingly, higher protein intake
has been shown to lower blood
pressure.

In a review of 40 controlled trials,
increased protein lowered systolic blood
pressure (the top number of a reading)
by 1.76 mm Hg on average and diastolic
blood pressure (the bottom number of a

reading) by 1.15 mm Hg. One study found that, in addition to lowering blood pressure, a high-protein diet also reduced LDL (bad) cholesterol and triglycerides.

SUMMARY Several studies note that higher protein intake can lower blood pressure. Some studies also demonstrate improvements in other risk factors for heart disease.

7. Helps Maintain Weight Loss

Because a high-protein diet boosts metabolism and leads to an automatic reduction in calorie intake and cravings, many people who increase their protein intake tend to lose weight almost instantly.

One study found that overweight women who ate 30% of their calories from protein lost 11 pounds (5 kg) in 12 weeks — though they didn't intentionally restrict their diet.

Protein also has benefits for fat loss during *intentional* calorie restriction.

In a 12-month study in 130 overweight people on a calorie-restricted diet, the high-protein group lost 53% more body fat than a normal-protein group eating the same number of calories. Of course, losing weight is just the beginning. Maintaining weight loss is a much greater challenge for most people.

A modest increase in protein intake has been shown to help with weight maintenance. In one study, increasing protein from 15% to 18% of calories reduced weight regain by 50%.

If you want to keep off excess weight, consider making a permanent increase in your protein intake.

SUMMARY Upping your protein intake can not only help you lose weight but keep it off in the long term.

8. Does Not Harm Healthy Kidneys

Many people wrongly believe that a high protein intake harms your kidneys.

It is true that restricting protein intake can benefit people with pre-existing kidney disease. This should not be taken lightly, as kidney problems can be very serious.

However, while high protein intake may harm individuals with kidney problems, it has no relevance to people with healthy kidneys. In fact, numerous studies underscore that high-protein diets have no harmful effects on people without kidney disease.

SUMMARY While protein can cause harm to people with kidney problems, it doesn't affect those with healthy kidneys.

9. Helps Your Body Repair Itself After Injury

Protein can help your body repair after it has been injured.

This makes perfect sense, as it forms the main building blocks of your tissues and organs.

Numerous studies demonstrate that eating more protein after injury can help speed up recovery.

SUMMARY Eating more protein can help you recover faster if you've been injured.

10. Helps You Stay Fit as You Age

One of the consequences of aging is that your muscles gradually weaken.

The most severe cases are referred to as age-related sarcopenia, which is one of the main causes of frailty, bone fractures, and reduced quality of life among older adults.

Eating more protein is one of the best ways to reduce age-related muscle deterioration and prevent sarcopenia.

Staying physically active is also crucial, and lifting weights or doing some sort of resistance exercise can work wonders.

SUMMARY Eating plenty of protein can help reduce the muscle loss associated with aging.

The Bottom Line

Even though a higher protein intake can have health benefits for many people, it is not necessary for everyone.

Most people already eat around 15% of their calories from protein, which is more than enough to prevent deficiency.

However, in certain cases, people can benefit from eating much more than that — up to 25–30% of calories.

If you need to lose weight, improve your metabolic health, or gain muscle mass and strength, make sure you're eating enough protein.

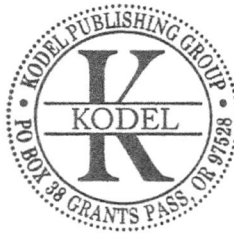

The Star Plan © 2017 – 2020

The Kodel Group, LLC

Echo Glenn

www.ingramcontent.com/pod-product-compliance
Lightning Source LLC
Chambersburg PA
CBHW050553280326
41933CB00011B/1832